Lemon Essential Oil

Benefits, Properties, Applications, Studies & Recipes

by Ann Sullivan

Published in USA by:

Ann Sullivan
217 N. Seacrest Blvd #9
Boynton Beach
FL 33425

© Copyright 2017

ISBN-13: ISBN-13: 978-1546505525
ISBN-10: 1546505520

Table of Contents

Introduction

What are essential oils, and how might they be used for therapeutic purposes?

Essential oils are ultra-potent oils, extracted from plants and flowers that have been utilized in medicine for centuries. Presently, they're most commonly used to supplement pharmaceutical medication, but they can also be an effective alternative to pharmaceuticals in the event that you don't have access to them. Before you dismiss essential oils as a means to support the body's natural defenses against injuries and illness, take a look at the historical evidence of the oils' medicinal competence in practice. Your average age-old medical text will demonstrate that essential oils, herbs, and plenty of other natural ingredients have, for thousands of years, successfully enhanced immune function to meet and defeat any number of ailments and injuries. Though traditional medicine is considered "alternative" now, it was once the gold standard. And, frankly, perhaps it still should be, as these natural age-tested remedies can fortify the body's battlements against everything from simple maladies, like headaches, cuts and bruises, to serious diseases, like cancer.

Essential oils are deemed "essential," because the oils are composed of the "essence" of the plant. The difference between essential oils and other oils – like olive oil or vegetable oil, for instance – is that essential oils have high volatility and reduced fixation, which results in faster evaporation, enabling their popular use in aromatherapy. Even at high temperatures, olive and vegetable oils don't evaporate.

Essential oils are especially necessary when it comes to a major natural or man-made disaster or some potential viral outbreak. In these types of dire situations, you may not have quick access (or any access at all) to your standard pharmaceutical supply; so essential oils, along with other alternative medicines, will be your go-to health aids in the case of social collapse, viral outbreak or devastating natural disaster. When medical access is null and void, alternatives to our modern-day standard are the only chance we have to keep pathogens at bay.

You probably don't realize that you already use essential oils every day. They're in perfumes, shampoos, soaps, ointments...they're even used in furniture polish. Why are they found in so many aromatic products? Well, basically, because essential oils are super concentrated aromatic liquids, so their scent is remarkably strong. Let's put this into perspective: to steam tea, you use a few leaves of peppermint or juniper; to produce a single ounce of essential oil, five whole *pounds* of peppermint or juniper leaves are required. Some sources claim that to produce twelve pounds of essential oil would necessitate an acre of peppermint, juniper, or any other oil you're looking to produce en masse. Unlike vegetable oil, you don't often find concentrated therapeutic-grade essential oils sold by the barrel; instead the oils are often sold in easily carried small, dark bottles, perfect for your GOOD bag (Get Out Of Dodge). Which is exactly what this book is aiming to help you do – get out of dodge with your most vital of essential oils intact, in particular a good supply of lemon essential oil.

Why lemon, you ask? Well, in order to get you quickly up to speed on this most essential of oils, below we've provided a condensed synopsis of lemon, after which we'll outline in greater detail the oil's history, properties, and common therapeutic uses, so that you – the consumer – might have a better understanding of the oil's benefits and applications. We've even provided supportive remedies for pure lemon, as well as blended recipes that incorporate the valuable oil. Chapter 3 will further detail past scientific research on lemon essential oil.

Now, let's get down to it – **Essential Oil 101: the Basics of Lemon.**

Summary: Lemon, or Citrus lemon, has traditionally been used for its cleaning and purifying properties and is believed to be native to Asia. As an antioxidant, lemon's composition is 68% d-limonene, which makes the oil an effective antidote to skin conditions. One kilo of oil is said to be made up of around 3,000 lemons. The highly concentrated oil serves as a tonic which may be used to support the nervous system. The vitamins and minerals available in this super fruit are more than can be found in any other, making lemon a powerful cleansing agent to rid the body of toxins.

Description: Lemon oil is commonly extracted by the cold pressed/expressed method. The citrus rind or peel is most often used. The oil is yellow in color, thin in consistency, and has a strong fresh lemon scent.

Uses: Beyond those applications previously mentioned, additional uses for lemon essential oil include supporting the body's natural defenses against athlete's foot, colds, flu, fever, chilblains, corns, oily or dull skin, warts, spots, varicose veins, insect repellant, allergies, asthma, constipation, hypertension, stomach ache, and sore throat. Lemon also serves as a cleanser, detoxifier and disinfectant, as well as in supporting the circulatory system. When it comes to mood and emotion, lemon essential oil calms and relieves stress, while uplifting and improving concentration

Properties: Antiviral, antibiotic, antioxidant, antifungal, antibacterial, antiseptic, immune stimulant, astringent, digestive tonic, diuretic, cleanser, and disinfectant.

Application: Dilute 1:1 with a carrier oil. You can apply topically, inhale directly, diffuse or use as a dietary supplement.

Safety Precautions: Lemon has been approved by the FDA for internal consumption and so can be used as a dietary supplement. However, If pregnant, breastfeeding or diabetic, consult your physician before using this oil. Lemon is also photosensitive, so if used topically, avoid direct sunlight for up to 24 hours. If you have sensitive skin, dilute heavily. Avoid using near fire or heat.

Fun facts: Lemon was called "median apple" by the Romans, who used the rind to scent clothing and repel insects. The Roman Goddess of Youth, Juventas, was symbolized by the fruit, perhaps due to its fresh scent and nature.

That sharp fresh scent also improves accuracy and mental acuity, according to a Japanese study which found that errors were reduced by 54% when the oil was diffused.

Chapter 1:
Benefits of Lemon Essential Oil

Lemon oil offers a number of therapeutic benefits; but you may be wondering what these benefits are. In this chapter, we'll take a closer look at the history of lemon and its many uses.

Cultivation of Lemon

Citrus limon is primarily obtained from the small Asian evergreen tree. The sour citrus fruit has long been used for culinary purposes, as well as medicinal ones. The whole fruit can be used – the pulp, the rind, and the juice – and each part possesses its own valuable properties. Citric acid makes up about 5-6% of the lemon's juice, which results in the strong sour taste, the strength of which allows lemon to play a prominent role in the food and drink industry.

A History of Lemon

The lemon tree's origin is uncertain. There is evidence, however, is that lemons were first cultivated in China, in northern Burma, and in the northeast Indian region of Assam. The origin of the word "lemon" is also uncertain, though it's believed to be Middle Eastern.

Eventually, lemons made their way to certain corners of the Middle East, arriving in Jerusalem. According to historical texts, they were featured during Jewish festivals around the 90s BC. Lemons were not referenced in European texts until the first century AD, when they were presented in Ancient Rome. Their presence expanded in the Middle East when they arrived in Iraq, Egypt and Persia around 700 AD. In Islamic gardens, lemons were used as ornamental plants, while the Arabic treatise on farming began to record the cultivation of lemons during the 10th century and the distribution throughout the Arab and Mediterranean regions expanded between 1000 and 1150 AD.

Still, it wasn't until the 15th century that lemons were significant in Europe, when they began to be cultivated in Genoa. Christopher Columbus is responsible for introducing the Americas to lemons when he brought the seeds to Hispaniola in 1493. The expansion was further exacerbated by the Spanish conquest in the New World, but the uses of the plant remained primarily ornamental and medicinal and, in fact, was used to cure seamen of scurvy. California and Florida saw more lemon cultivation during the 19th century.

Versatility

Throughout its existence, lemon has grown into one of the most versatile fruits known to man. As mentioned, a vast variety of food and drinks incorporate lemon zest, rind and juice. Drinks which incorporate lemon include cocktails, soft drinks, tea, and lemonade, while foods include marinades for fish, marmalade, puddings, rice, and many baked goods. The oil also offers other foods its preservative properties and so is used to preserve in the short-term those produce which oxidize quickly, such as bananas, apples, and avocados.

But the benefits of lemon don't stop at food. Lemon can also be used in cleaning, as the oil and the juice have the ability to disinfect, deodorize, bleach, and eliminate grease. A lemon's acid helps to fight tough stains through its easy dissolution and abrasivity. The oil can also be used as an insecticide.

And, medicinally, the properties of lemon are extraordinary, but we'll get to those properties later in the chapter.

Chemical Components

In order to generate the essential oil from the lemon, the rind must be cold pressed or expressed. This results in the oil's key chemical components, which are primarily camphene, a-pinene, b-pinene, myrcene, linalool, limonene, sabinene, a-terpinene, b-bisabolene, trans-a-bergamotene, neral and nerol.

Main Properties of Lemon Essential Oil

Along with the properties previously mentioned in the introduction, lemon oil possesses antiviral, antibiotic, antioxidant, antibacterial, antifungal, antiseptic, immune stimulant, astringent, digestive tonic, diuretic, carminative, cleanser, and disinfectant properties. With such a versatile range, lemon is well equipped to fight off any pathogen in the body's path.

Lemon, as mentioned, is composed of many natural chemicals, among them linalool and limonene. These components are what instill the enormously beneficial properties within lemon essential oil. We'll outline these properties below.

Disinfectant & Cleanser

The fact that lemon is added to so many household cleaners doesn't come down to the fresh scent alone; being a disinfectant, lemon is the ultimate cleaning agent, because it eliminates contamination. As mentioned previously, lemon also deodorizes, bleaches, and destroys grease, and so can be used to clean dishes, clothing, and practically any surface.

Diuretic

If you're looking to lose water weight and reduce blood pressure, lemon essential oil is your agent. The oil stimulates urination, promoting not only the loss of water weight, but the loss of fats, uric acid, sodium, and other body toxins.

Carminative

By administrationing excess gas build up and/or removing it from the intestines, lemon essential oil provides relief from abdominal pain, excess sweating, and uncomfortable indigestion.

Antioxidant

Anything high in antioxidants – whether fruit, beans, or essential oils – is a powerful advocate for your body. Antioxidants both protect against free radicals and repair their damage. What are free radicals? Free radicals are destructive chemicals that invade your body, produced by substances both inside and out. Some free radicals (or oxidants) form through normal bodily reactions, like inflammation, metabolism and aerobic respiration. Other free radicals form outside the body, but enter it due to exposure. These include harmful pollutants, toxins, smoking, drinking alcohol, X-rays, and UV rays, to name a few. Although our bodies produce their own antioxidants, these often become damaged as we grow older; thus, introducing antioxidants into our bodies allows these nutrients and enzymes to assist in chemical reactions which destroy the oxidants or free radicals. Lemon essential oil is a moderate antioxidant, aiming to detox the body of free radicals that lead to disease.

Antibacterial

Lemon's antibacterial properties make it a powerful protectant against diseases produced by bacteria, such as skin issues and infections, like urinary tract or colon infections. It can even combat cholera, typhoid and food poisoning. What's great is that, unlike some prescription drugs, lemon has no ill effects on bodily health or on the healthy natural flora that exists within the stomach and intestines.

Antifungal

While bacteria and viruses are plenty evil, fungi commonly lead to the most deadly infections, whether external or internal. Your ears, throat and nose are the most likely to become infected by fungi, the infections of which can be both excruciating and unsightly. If left untreated, fungal infections can kill, as they may spread to the brain. Lemon essential oil protects against these infections and more and is particularly effective against skin infections.

Antiviral

The antiviral protection that lemon essential oil grants will essentially empower the immune system, building up a tougher wall of security that most colds, measles or mumps are unlikely to scale. By boosting white blood cell count and function, this immune stimulant will ensure that your body is better prepared to protect against deadly viral infections.

Antiseptic

The antiseptic and disinfectant properties of lemon essential oil can be reaped topically, applied directly to wounds, or even through burning; the smoke from the oil may help destroy airborne germs. Internal use will help keep wounds from becoming infections, while external use will help stave off tetanus.

Astringent

For those who do not know what an astringent is, it's a chemical compound that shrinks body tissues, which means it can aid skin issues and irritations, everything from acne to insect bites. The astringent property of lemon essential oil benefits everything from skin to hair to gums to muscles to intestines. As an astringent, lemon is an anti-agent, combatting muscle loss through the ability to strengthen. This astringent and coagulant properties also mean that diarrhea can be relieved through use of lemon essential oil, as well as wound and cut bleeding.

Digestive

By boosting the production of absorptive enzymes, the digestibility of nutrients, and the secretion of digestive juices, lemon essential oil aids the digestive tract significantly, which can make a great impact on your overall health by increasing those nutrients you absorb from food.

Common Medicinal Uses

Citrus lemon has traditionally been used for its cleaning and purifying properties and, as an antioxidant with 68% d-limonene, lemon essential oil an effective antidote for skin conditions. The highly concentrated oil serves as a tonic which may be used to support the nervous system. The vitamins and minerals available in this super fruit are more than can be found in any other, making lemon a powerful cleansing agent to rid the body of toxins. Let's take a look at some of the oil's primary medicinal uses.

Skin Care

Nothing beats lemon essential oil when it comes to lackluster skin. The oil's astringent properties invigorate dull skin, while its detoxifying properties help cleanse and eliminate excess oil. Whether using lemon essential oil to defy skin aging or to reduce adolescent skin issues, like pimples and acne, the antiseptic and astringent properties are the best, bar none.

Immune System

The vitamin content in lemon essential oil is what makes it such a superb immune system support. Lemon essential oil also boosts circulation and increases white blood cell count. By doing so, this immune stimulant will ensure that your body is better prepared to protect against deadly viral infections.

Stomach Issues

As a carminative, lemon essential oil is beneficial when it comes to stomach issues. Whether you have menstrual cramps, indigestion, nausea or upset stomach, a dosage of this oil will help ease the pain and uncomfortable nature of these issues.

Stress

Ever wonder why school and office environments are often scented with lemon? It's no accident. The scent of lemon has been shown to be calming and also increase alertness and focus. It eases anxiety, mental fatigue, nervousness, and exhaustion. If you're feeling stressed, you can combat your negative emotions or keep them from developing through essential oil administration, whether aromatherapeutic, ingestion, or topical.

Asthma

The inhalation of lemon essential oil helps to promote breathing and respiratory airflow by clearing sinuses and nasal passages. In this way, it's been shown to be useful in supporting the body's natural defenses against asthma and other respiratory issues.

Infectious Diseases

Lemon essential oil is also a good combatant against infectious diseases, such as typhoid and malaria. It has the ability to control fevers which sometimes accompany these infections.

Insomnia

The calming effect of lemon essential oil can help the body relax and can ease the sleepless into sleep. Those suffering from insomnia should diffuse lemon essential oil in their bedroom or place a drop or two on their linens.

Hair Care

Lemon essential oil invokes strength, health, and shine in the hair, and so is often used as a hair tonic. The oil also effectively combats dandruff, so a drop or two in your shampoo should eliminate this issue.

Weight Management

A drop or two of essential oil at every meal and in every drink has been shown to satisfy the appetite and keep from overeating. As a diuretic, it also stimulates urination, promoting not only the loss of water weight, but the loss of fats, uric acid, sodium, and other body toxins.

Safety Precautions & Common Applications

Safety

Some adverse effects may evolve when using pure essential oils. Some essential oils should not be used when pregnant, for example, as they may cause miscarriage. Allergic reactions, too, may occur, especially when applied topically. Always administer an allergy test before committing fully to topical application. When used with other medications, essential oils may react negatively. If you are on any current prescription medications or have a chronic illness, such as high blood pressure, epilepsy or liver disease, then researching the effects of essential oils against your own personal medical history will eliminate any potentially problematic issues.

Lemon essential oil has been approved by the FDA for internal consumption and so can be used as a dietary supplement. However, If pregnant, breastfeeding or diabetic, consult your physician before using this oil. Lemon is also photosensitive, so if used topically, avoid direct sunlight for up to 24 hours. If you have sensitive skin, dilute heavily. Avoid using near fire or heat.

Blends

Oftentimes, essential oils are manufactured as blends of several pure oils. For instance, Protective Essential Oil Blend *(See EverythingEssential.com for Blend Recipe)* is a mix of cinnamon, clove, rosemary, and eucalyptus. This blend can be used to boost the immune system to help support the body's defenses against colds, viruses and flus. The downside to blends is that the more oils added to the mix, the higher the probability your patient may react negatively to the blend if he/she is prone to allergies. There is also the possibility of phototoxicity when working with blends.

Regardless of these possible effects, essential oils are a viable option for support the body's defenses against a number of conditions. Those looking to enhance the maintenance of their own personal health, or that of their family, should become educated on the uses of essential oils, their natural remedies and the methods of application. Only then can you begin building your kit of essential oils for survival.

Chapter 2:
Recipes for Lemon Essential Oil

In this chapter, we'll offer various recipes for lemon essential oil, both for pure lemon supportive remedies and for blends which incorporate the oil. For pure supportive remedies, we've provided the appropriate application and dosage to target specific ailments, from air pollution to tonsillitis. When it comes to blends, herbalists and aromatherapists often combine lemon essential oil with ylang ylang, lavender, rose, sandalwood, neroli, tea tree or geranium essential oils. We'll offer some fantastic supportive blending options in the second half of this chapter.

Pure Supportive Remedies

Air Pollution

If your home's locale offers low air quality, diffuse lemon essential oil throughout. You can also diffuse after painting to combat fumes.

Anxiety

To relieve anxiety, place one drop of lemon essential oil into your palm and rub your hands together. Place your hand over your nose and mouth and inhale. You can also diffuse throughout your home to relieve tension and stress.

Atherosclerosis

Combat atherosclerosis by diluting lemon essential oil in a 1:1 ratio with a carrier oil and massaging into the chest. You can also diffuse throughout your home.

Bites/Stings

To relieve pain, combat infection, and promote quick healing, dilute lemon essential oil in a 1:1 ratio with a carrier oil and place on the affected sting or bite.

Blood Pressure

Regulate blood pressure by adding a single drop of lemon essential oil to your tea or water. Take three times a day.

Brain Injury

Support the body's natural defenses against brain injuries by diffusing lemon essential oil throughout the room. You can also place a drop on the patient's shirt collar or pillow or you can dilute lemon essential oil in a 1:1 ratio with a carrier oil and massage into scalp, neck and shoulders.

Cold Sores

To eliminate or stave off cold sores, dilute lemon essential oil in a 1:1 ratio with a carrier oil and dab directly onto the cold sore or apply as a supportive lip balm.

Colds

Combat colds by diffusing lemon essential oil throughout the home or place several drops in your wet laundry before drying. You can also apply topically by diluting lemon essential oil in a 1:1 ratio with a carrier oil and massaging into the chest.

Concentration

This is especially great for teachers. If you want to stimulate concentration and focus for study or work, place a drop of lemon essential oil on your shirt collar or diffuse throughout the room.

Constipation

To relieve constipation, dilute lemon essential oil in a 1:5 ratio with coconut oil and massage in a clockwise motion over the abdomen.

Depression

Combat depression by placing a drop on your pillow or in your water or tea. You can also diffuse throughout the room or dilute the oil in a 1:1 ratio with a carrier oil and apply topically, massaging into scalp, neck and shoulders.

Digestion

To aid digestion, place a drop in your drinking water or incorporate into your cooking. You can also apply topically by diluting lemon essential oil in a 1:1 ratio with a carrier oil and massaging it into the abdomen.

Disinfectant

Use lemon essential oil as a disinfectant throughout your home. Place a drop in your dishwater, a drop in your natural household cleaners, a drop in your laundry. You can also put three drops in your bathwater or dilute lemon essential oil in a 1:1 ratio with a carrier oil and apply topically in a full-body massage.

Dry Throat

Eliminate dry throat by placing a drop of lemon essential oil into your drinking water. You can also try combining the oil with sea salts and warm water for a gargling solution.

Dysentery

Target dysentery by diluting lemon essential oil in a 1:1

ratio with a carrier oil and massaging it into the lower abdomen and lower back, over the area of the intestines.

Energizing

Give yourself a boost of energy by diluting lemon essential oil in a 1:1 ratio with a carrier oil and massaging it into the chest and neck, and into the reflex points on the hands and feet. You can also place a drop in your drinking water for immediate energy.

Fever

To reduce or regulate fever, dilute lemon essential oil in a 1:5 ratio with a carrier oil and massage into forehead, neck, shoulders, and inside ears. You can also place a drop into cool drinking fluids.

Flu

Support the body's natural defenses against the flu by diluting lemon essential oil in a 1:1 ratio with a carrier oil and massaging it over aches and pains, into the abdomen, and into the reflex points on your hands and feet. You can also place a drop on the pillow of the sickbed and diffuse throughout the home.

Gout

Target gout by diluting lemon essential oil in a 1:1 ratio with a carrier oil and applying to the infected area, or you can add a few drops of the oil to warm water and allow the infected area to soak. You can also take orally by placing a drop of oil into a teaspoon of honey and ingesting 2-5 times daily.

Hangovers

Need a quick hangover fix? Dilute lemon essential oil in a 1:1 ratio with a carrier oil and massage it into the abdomen, chest, and the reflex points on your hands and feet. You can also simply inhale directly, add a drop to drinking water, or place a few drops in your bathwater.

Heartburn

Relieve heartburn by diluting lemon essential oil in a 1:1 ratio with a carrier oil and massaging it in a downward motion from throat to stomach, as well as across the arches and soles of the feet.

Intestinal Parasites

Rid of intestinal parasites by diluting lemon essential oil in a 1:1 ratio with a carrier oil and massaging it into the abdomen and the soles of the feet. You can also add a drop to your drinking water.

Kidney Stones

To target kidney stones, place a drop of lemon essential oil in each meal or into your drinking water.

Lymphatic Cleansing

Cleanse your lymphatic system by diluting lemon essential oil in a 1:1 ratio with a carrier oil and massaging it into your body, working from your extremities toward the heart. You can also diffuse throughout the home.

MRSA

Combat MRSA by diluting lemon essential oil in a 1:1 ratio with a carrier oil and applying topically in a full-body massage.

Oily Hair

To reduce oily hair, place a drop of lemon essential oil into your shampoo or dilute 3-4 drops with water in a 1:3 ratio and massage directly into your scalp every time you wash your hair. You can also take orally with drinking water to stimulate internal health for hair growth.

Overeating

Keep from overeating by diffusing lemon essential oil throughout the home. You can also put a drop on your shirt collar or place a drop in your palms, rub your hands together, and run them through your hair.

Pancreatitis

Combat pancreatitis by diluting lemon essential oil in a 1:1 ratio with a carrier oil and massaging it into the hands and feet. You can also inhale directly, diffuse throughout the home, or add a drop to your drinking water.

Postpartum Depression

To relieve postpartum depression, diffuse lemon essential oil throughout the home. You can also put a drop on your shirt collar or place a drop in your palms, rub your hands together, and run them through your hair.

Skin

Use lemon essential oil as a skin toner by diluting the oil in a 1:5 ratio with purified water. Place the oil/water combo in a spray bottle and spritz on the face. Do not spray directly into eyes.

Stress

Combat stress by steaming two drops of lemon essential oil in a pan of water, remove the steaming pan from the stove, pour into a bowl, place a towel over your head and inhale. If you don't feel it's done its job the first time, you can reheat that same water and use it once more without adding more oil. You can also place a drop onto your shirt collar for portable stress relief.

Throat Infection

Strengthen the body's natural defenses against throat infections by diluting lemon essential oil in a 1:1 ratio with a carrier oil and applying topically in a full-body massage. You can also diffuse throughout the home or combine the oil with sea salts and warm water for a gargling solution.

Tonsillitis

Eliminate tonsillitis by diluting lemon essential oil in a 1:1 ratio with a carrier oil and applying topically in a full-body massage. You can also diffuse throughout the home or combine the oil with sea salts and warm water for a gargling solution.

Varicose Veins

Reduce the appearance of varicose veins by diluting lemon essential oil in a 1:1 ratio with a carrier oil and applying topically in an upwards stroke towards the heart.

Water Purification

To purify water, place a drop of lemon essential oil in a glass of water. Mix well and then allow to rest for 5 minutes. Then drink up!

Blends

Acne Serum

Ingredients

- 3 drops Lemon Essential Oil
- 3 drops Lavender Essential Oil
- 3 drops Frankincense Essential Oil
- 1 Tbsp Jojoba Oil

Directions

Combine all ingredients in a glass jar or dropper bottle. Place the lid on and shake vigorously to combine. After washing the face with water every night, apply 2-3 drops of the serum, massaging into the skin in a circular motion. Shake well before each use.

Antiseptic Ointment

Ingredients

- 10 drops Lemon Essential Oil
- 20 drops Lavender Essential Oil
- 50 drops Tea Tree Essential Oil
- 1 cup Carrier Oil (Olive or Almond Oil recommended)
- 1 ½ ounces Beeswax (grated)
- ¼ tsp Vitamin E Oil

Directions

Fill a saucepan with 1 inch of water. Add the grated beeswax to a mason jar and place in the saucepan. Over low-medium heat, stir the beeswax until melted. Remove from heat. Allow the beeswax to cool slightly before mixing in remaining ingredients. Stir until well combined. Apply to wounds, cuts and stings. Shake well before each use.

Allergies

Ingredients

- 2 drops Peppermint Essential Oil
- 2 drops Lemon Essential Oil
- 2 drops Lavender Essential Oil
- 8 ounce Water

Directions

Combine all ingredients in an 8 ounce glass of drinking water, and drink three times a day – morning, noon and night.

Chest Congestion

Ingredients

- 1 drop Cinnamon Essential Oil
- 1 drop Lemon Essential Oil
- 1 tsp Carrier Oil

Directions

To clear up chest congestion, combine all ingredients and massage into your chest three times a day.

Digestive Blend

Ingredients

- 6 drops Lemon Essential Oil
- 6 drops Peppermint Essential Oil

Directions

To aid digestion, place all ingredients into a "00" capsule, and ingest 1 capsule daily.

Eye Cream

Ingredients

- 1 ounce Coconut Oil
- 2 drops Lemon Essential Oil
- 2 drops Frankincense Essential Oil
- 2 drops Lavender Essential Oil

Directions

Combine all ingredients in a small glass jar. To reduce fine lines and wrinkles, apply topically to the eye area. Avoid putting directly in the eye.

Focus

Ingredients

- 2 drops Frankincense Essential Oil
- 2 drops Lemon Essential Oil

Directions

To sharpen focus, steam two drops each of frankincense and lemon essential oils in a pan of water, remove the steaming pan from the stove, pour into a bowl, place a towel over your head and inhale.

Protective Blend Oil

Ingredients

- 10 drops Rosemary Essential Oil
- 15 drops Eucalyptus Essential Oil
- 20 drops Cinnamon Bark Essential Oil
- 35 drops Lemon Essential Oil
- 40 drops Clove Bud Essential Oil
- 12 ounces Distilled Water

Directions

Combine all ingredients in a dark colored glass spray bottle and, during cold and flu season or if there's illness in the house, spray in all rooms to stimulate the immune system. You can also dilute the homemade protective blend with a carrier oil and apply to the soles of the feet.

Gluten Intolerance

Ingredients

- 1 drop Cinnamon Bark Essential Oil
- 2 drops Grapefruit Essential Oil
- 2 drops Ginger Essential Oil
- 2 drops Lemon Essential Oil

Instructions

To help target gluten intolerance, place all ingredients into a "00" capsule, and ingest 1 capsule a day.

Healing Salve

Ingredients

- 4 Tbsp Beeswax
- 1 cup Extra Virgin Olive Oil
- 1 cup Virgin Coconut Oil
- 2 tsp Vitamin E Oil (divided
- 40 drops Lavender Essential Oil (divided)
- 32 drops Lemon Essential Oil (divided)
- 24 drops Tea Tree Essential Oil (divided)

Directions

Combine beeswax, coconut oil and olive oil in a mason jar and place jar in a saucepan with 1 inch of water. Over medium-low heat, mix until melted and well blended. Remove from the stove and add in the essential oils, mixing until combined. In four separate 4 ounce glass jars, divide up the essential oils equally (10 drops lavender, 8 drops lemon, 6 drops tea tree, ½ tsp vitamin E oil per jar). In the jars, pour in equal amounts of the beeswax-oil combo. Let cool completely before use. To apply, rub over wounds, cuts, or stings.

Libido

Ingredients

- 6 drops Lemon Essential Oil
- 6 drops Ylang Ylang Essential Oil

Directions

To stimulate the libido, place all ingredients into a "00" capsule, and ingest 1 capsule daily.

Mental Clarity

Ingredients

- 6 drops Lemon Essential Oil
- 4 drops Rosemary Essential Oil
- 2 drops Cypress Essential Oil
- 1 tsp Carrier Oil

Directions

To clarify the mind, combine all ingredients and apply topically, massaging into temples and into the soles of your feet.

Mood Stabilizer

Ingredients

- 2 drops Lemon Essential Oil
- 2 drops Geranium Essential Oil

Directions

To stabilize your mood, diffuse the oils and deeply breathe in the vapors.

Refresher

Ingredients

- 2 drops Lemon Essential Oil
- 2 drops Eucalyptus Essential Oil

Directions

To feel refreshed, steam two drops each of eucalyptus and lemon essential oils in a pan of water, remove the steaming pan from the stove, pour into a bowl, place a towel over your head and inhale.

Sore Throat Spray

Ingredients

- 15 drops Four Thieves Essential Oil
- 5 drops Lemon Essential Oil
- 1/8 ounce Vodka
- 1 ½ ounces Purified Water
- 2 tsp Raw Honey

Directions

Combine ingredients in a spray bottle. Place the lid on and shake well. To apply, spray 1-2 squirts in the back of the throat, shaking well before each use.

Vapor Rub

Ingredients

- 3 drops Lemon Essential Oil
- 3 drops Peppermint Essential Oil
- 6 drops Eucalyptus Essential Oil
- 1 Tbsp Coconut Oil

Directions

Combine all ingredients in a small bowl, mixing thoroughly. Apply topically, massaging into chest, back, and neck.

Chapter 3:
Lemon Essential Oil Studies

Many studies have been done on essential oils to discover and prove their therapeutic qualities. In the case of the great number of lemon studies, many of the properties attributed to the essential oil (noted in this book and elsewhere) are quite often validated through the scientific research of accredited universities and published by accredited scientific journals. In this chapter, we'll discuss a small portion of these studies. It's important to note that research on essential oils is constant and evolving. Keep up with any recent research, as it may turn up even further valuable uses of these miracle oils.

Study 1 – Antifungal Properties

In this study published by Mycopathologia, the antifungal effects of lemon essential oil were examined, with the following results: "This study addresses the chemical composition of some commercial lemon essential oils and their antifungal potential against selected Candida yeast strains. Antifungal potential and minimum inhibitory concentrations were determined for six commercial lemon essential oils against five Candida yeast strains (Candida albicans 31, Candida tropicalis 32, Candida glabrata 33, Candida glabrata 35 and Candida glabrata 38)... Our study characterises lemon essential oils, which could be used as very effective natural remedies against candidiasis caused by C. albicans."

As noted, the study examined the effect of lemon essential oil on five different Candida strains. Let's take a look at each of these strains. The first two strains of fungi, Candida albicans and Candida tropicalis, develop as yeast and filamentous cells, and can potentially cause genital and oral infections. Candida albicans also increases the probability of mortality in immunocompromised individuals (cancer or AIDS patients, for instance). The last three Candida strains tested, Candida glabrata 33, 35 and 38, are non-dimorphic yeasts which have the potential to become pathogens in the urogenital tract and the bloodstream of immunocompromised individuals, especially in the elderly and those with HIV.

The study showed that lemon essential oil was an active combatant against these five Candida strains, which demonstrates its antifungal properties.

Reference
http://www.ncbi.nlm.nih.gov/pubmed/24436010

http://www.ncbi.nlm.nih.gov/pmc/articles/PMC3915084/pdf/11046_2013_Article_9723.pdf]

Study 2 – Nausea

In this study published by the Iran Red Crescent Medical Journal, the anti-nausea effects of lemon essential oil were examined, with the following results: "Nausea and vomiting of pregnancy are amongst the most common complaints that effects on both the physical and mental conditions of the pregnant women. Due to the increasing tendency of women to use herbal medications during pregnancy, the effect of lemon inhalation aromatherapy on nausea and vomiting of pregnancy was investigated in this study...There was a statistically significant difference between the two groups in the mean scores of nausea and vomiting on the second and fourth days ($P = 0.017$ and $P = 0.039$, respectively). The means of nausea and vomiting intensity in the second and fourth days in the intervention group were significantly lower than the control group. In addition, in intragroup comparison with ANOVA with repeated measures, the nausea and vomiting mean in the five intervals, showed a statistically significant difference in each group ($P < 0.001$ and $P = 0.049$, respectively)."

After comparing a control group of pregnant women with a test group receiving lemon essential oil aromatherapy, this study found that those in the test group experienced a significant reduction in morning sickness. Particularly in the second and fourth days of the trial, nausea and vomiting were markedly reduced in the test group. This demonstrates the effectiveness of lemon essential oil in its ability to control or reduce nausea and vomiting.

Reference
http://www.ncbi.nlm.nih.gov/pubmed/24829772

http://www.ncbi.nlm.nih.gov/pmc/articles/PMC4005434/
pdf/ircmj-16-14360.pdf]

Study 3 – Insecticide

In this study published by the Journal of Insect Science, the insecticidal effects of lemon essential oil were examined, with the following results: "The vine mealybug, Planococcus ficus (Signoret) (Hemiptera: Pseudococcidae), is a pest in grape vine growing areas worldwide. The essential oils from the following aromatic plants were tested for their insecticidal activity against P. Ficus...lemon, Citrus limon L. ...The essential oils from citrus, peppermint and thyme leaved savory were more or equally toxic compared to the reference product... No phytotoxic symptoms were observed on grape leaves treated with the citrus essential oils."

This study tested lemon essential oil, along with other essential oils, against the vine mealybug, Planococcus ficus, which affects grapevines worldwide, particularly in South Africa. In the US, P. Ficus is endemic in California grape vines. Lemon essential oil showed equal insecticidal activity against the P.Ficus as the reference product, which was paraffin oil. The use of lemon essential oil also did not result in phytotoxicity, a toxic effect which damages plant growth. The research demonstrates lemon essential oil's potential use as an insecticide.

Reference & Photo Credit:
http://www.ncbi.nlm.nih.gov/pubmed/24766523]

http://www.ncbi.nlm.nih.gov/pmc/articles/PMC4015406/pdf/031.013.14201.pdf]

Study 4 – Antibacterial Properties

In this study published by the Brazilian Journal of Microbiology, the antibacterial effects of lemon essential oil were examined, with the following results: "Alicyclobacillus acidoterrestris is considered to be one of the important target microorganisms in the quality control of acidic canned foods. There is an urgent need to develop a suitable method for inhibiting or controlling the germination and outgrowth of A.acidoterrestris in acidic drinks. The aim of this work was to evaluate the chemicals used in the lemon industry (sodium benzoate, potassium sorbate), and lemon essential oil as a natural compound, against a strain of A.acidoterrestris in MEB medium and in lemon juice concentrate...The results pointed out that sodium benzoate (500-1000-2000 ppm) and lemon essential oil (0.08-0.12-0.16%) completely inhibited the germination of A. acidoterrestris spores in MEB medium and LJC for 11 days."

Alicyclobacillus acidoterrestris is a Gram positive, sporeforming bacteria, which is able to survive pasteurization procedures in the canning industry and grow in products, causing spoilage. A. acidoterrestris has become the bar when designing pasteurization processes for highly acid foods, so the fact that lemon essential oil showed complete inhibition of A. acidoterrestris germination is a brilliant outcome for the canning industry.

Reference

http://www.ncbi.nlm.nih.gov/pubmed/24688502

http://www.ncbi.nlm.nih.gov/pmc/articles/PMC3958178/pdf/bmj-44-4-1133.pdf]

Study 5 – Antioxidant Properties

In this study published by Journal of Oleo Science, the antifungal effects of lemon essential oil were examined, with the following results: "This study sought to investigate the effects of essential oil from lemon (Citrus limon) peels on acetylcholinesterase (AChE) and butyrylcholinesterase (BChE) activities in vitro... The inhibition of AChE and BChE activities, inhibition of pro-oxidant induced lipid peroxidation and antioxidant activities could be possible mechanisms for the use of the essential oil in the management and prevention of oxidative stress-induced neurodegeneration."

By testing lemon essential oil against acetylcholinesterase and butyrylcholinesterase, both of which are enzymes which actively terminate neurotransmission, the study found that lemon essential oil inhibits the damaging activity of these enzymes. This, alongside the oil's antioxidant properties, means that lemon essential oil may have the potential to support the body's natural defenses against neurodegenerative diseases, such as Alzheimer's, ALS, Huntington's, or Parkinson's.

Reference & Photo Credit:
http://www.ncbi.nlm.nih.gov/pubmed/24599102

https://www.jstage.jst.go.jp/article/jos/63/4/63_ess13166
/_pdf

Study 6 – Antioxidant Properties

In this study published by the Journal of Biomedicine and
Biotechnology, the antioxidant effects of lemon essential oil
were examined, with the following results: "The antioxidant
and antinociceptive activities of Citrus limon essential oil
(EO) were assessed in mice or in vitro tests...EO possesses
a strong antioxidant potential according to the scavenging
assays. Moreover, it presented scavenger activity against all
in vitro tests. Orally, EO (50, 100, and 150 mg/kg)
significantly reduced the number of writhes, and, at highest
doses, it reduced the number of paw licks. Whereas
naloxone antagonized the antinociceptive action of EO
(highest doses), this suggested, at least, the participation of
the opioid system."

Again, in this study, the antioxidant properties of lemon
essential oil were found to be strong. Furthermore, the
antinociceptive activity of the oil was examined.
Nociception relates to the processing of harmful stimuli in
the nervous system, which is directed to the body's "pain
receptors" or, in other words, its ability to sense bodily
pain. Lemon essential oil was found to have antinociceptive

properties, which indicates that it can be used to reduce and relieve pain sensitivity.

Reference

http://www.ncbi.nlm.nih.gov/pubmed/21660140]

http://www.ncbi.nlm.nih.gov/pmc/articles/PMC3110330/pdf/JBB2011-678673.pdf]

Study 7 – Cross Contamination

In this study published by the Poultry Science Association, the anti-cross-contaminant effects of lemon essential oil were examined, with the following results: "The objectives of this study were to determine the effect of an essential oil blend (EO; carvacrol, thymol, eucalyptol, lemon) administered in drinking water on the performance, mortality, water consumption, pH of crop and ceca, and Salmonella enterica serovar Heidelberg fecal shedding and colonization in broiler birds following Salmonella Heidelberg challenge and feed withdrawal...The EO used in the study may control Salmonella Heidelberg contamination in crops of broilers when administered in drinking water and therefore may reduce the potential for cross-contamination of the carcass when the birds are processed."

Another important health issue in the food industry is

cross-contamination. This study analyzed the efficacy of an essential oil blend which included lemon on the inhibition of Salmonella Heidelberg, a contaminant in crops. Applying the blend to the broiler birds' drinking water reduced the rate of cross-contamination.

Reference & Photo Credit:
http://www.ncbi.nlm.nih.gov/pubmed/23436536]

http://ps.oxfordjournals.org/content/92/3/836.full.pdf+html]

Study 8 – Oral Hygiene

In this study published by the J Food Sci Technol, the oral hygienic effects of lemon essential oil were examined, with the following results: "We have isolated 4 antibacterial substances that were active against the oral bacteria that cause dental caries and periodontitis, such as Streptococcus mutans, Prevotella intermedia, and Porphyromonas gingivalis, from lemon peel, a waste product in the citrus industry...Among these, 8-Geranyloxypsolaren, 5-geranyloxypsolaren, and 5-geranyloxy-7-methoxycoumarin exhibited high antibacterial activity... Further, the above 3 compounds were present in lemon essential oil and abundantly present in the residue produced upon the cooling treatment of concentrated lemon essential oil."

Streptococcus mutans is an oral bacteria which causes

cavities and tooth decay, Prevotella intermedia causes gingivitis and periodontitis, and Porphyromonas gingivalis forms black colonies on blood agar and is found, not only in the oral cavity, but in the upper gastrointestinal tract, the colon, and the respiratory tract. Three of the compounds present in lemon essential oil demonstrated high antibacterial activity against these oral bacterial strains.

Reference
http://www.ncbi.nlm.nih.gov/pubmed/23572799]

http://www.ncbi.nlm.nih.gov/pmc/articles/PMC3551 112/pdf/13197_2011_Article_330.pdf]

Chapter 4:
The Ins & Outs of Essential Oils

Where do essential oils come from?

Plants and plant species naturally produce essential oils for various reasons; one being to draw pollinator insects to them, another being to repel invading organisms (bacteria, animals). A number of chemical compounds compose each plant's essential oil, and the combination of these compounds are specific to each oil, which then instills in the oil its own unique properties. Essential oils can be harnessed from all sorts of plant components, including flowers, leaves, bark, fruit, roots, and resin. For instance, cinnamon oil is harnessed from bark, lemon oil from the peel, and lavender oil from lavender flowers. Certain plants can produce a few chemical variants of the same essential oil, which are acquired from different parts of the plant. Some of these parts produce a large amount of oil, while others produce just a smidgen. The oil's quality and potency depends upon a number of factors, including the subspecies of the plant, its soil conditions, the time of year, and even the time of day you harvest it.

How are essential oils extracted?

Essential oils can be extracted from plants through various methods, including pressing, distillation, solvent, and maceration. Let's take a brief look at each:

Pressing Method

Commonly used with citrus fruit, the pressing method extracts the oil through a technique which involves pushing the fruit peels through a press. Oily fruits and plants are best suited for this technique. Orange oil, for example, is extracted from orange skins through the pressing method.

Distillation Method

This technique harkens back to the days of moonshiners, as the same sort of method used to create strong liquor can be used to extract essential oils. Using a still, boiled water, and plant materials, will create steam which is then cooled by coils and condensed into a combination of water and oil. This combination does not mix, so the oil can then be extracted from it.

Solvent Method

Through a multi-step process, certain plant and flower oils can be extracted using alcohol and other solvents, which extort the essential oil from the plant materials.

Maceration Method

When a "carrier," fixed oil, or lard is mixed with the plant material and set out in the sun over a period of time, the carrier oil is infused with the plant's essence. Heat sources, other than the sun, are often used to speed the process. Throughout the process more plant material is added to produce a more potent oil.

How do you use essential oils?

Although some studies about the effectiveness of essential oils are conducted by small companies or even individuals, a number of them are conducted by the food and cosmetic industries. In general, the pharmaceutical industry shows next to no interest in herbal medicine, primarily because there are few options to patent such products. As such, the product's lack of profitability results in a lack of research funding. Regardless, the historical uses of essential oils tell us what we need to know: these oils have been effectively administered for centuries. The therapeutic qualifications of essential oils can be plotted in the survival of the human race across cultures and generations.

Another reason that studies on essential oils have not resulted in much conclusive evidence as to their overall effectiveness is because definitive results are sometimes difficult to prove, as the quality of each batch of oil can vary for a number of reasons. One is that essential oils are impossible to standardize. As mentioned above, even the slightest variance in soil conditions and the time of harvesting – as well as innumerable other factors – will produce a different product quality and potency. In addition, essential oils are often obtained from various species of the same plant; Eucalyptus radiata and Eucalyptus globulus can both be used in the making of therapeutic-grade eucalyptus oil and as a result, they may have slightly different properties and degrees of strength or effectiveness.

Just as there are a number of methods by which to extract essential oils, there are a number of methods to administer them therapeutically. The variety of chemical compounds in each essential oil means that their benefits and applications also vary across the board. Below are a few of these methods.

Topical Administration

Direct application of many essential oils works like a sponge, as skin absorbs chemicals and other things (like sunlight, for instance). Topical application is best when you want to clear up an ailment on the skin's surface, or in the underlying muscle tissue. When applying topically, you may either massage the oil into the skin, or simply dab on the skin for therapeutic results. You might combine the essential oil with a carrier oil for topical use in order to dilute its potency. This is safer, as the oil is concentrated. You may support your body's defenses against rash or muscle pain in this manner, but you should always test your patient for allergies before applying. Adverse effects are produced by natural chemicals as much as synthetic ones; poison ivy, for example.

To test for allergens, place a drop or two on your patient's inner forearm. If a rash develops within 12 to 24 hours, then the patient is allergic. In addition, phototoxicity – sun exposure resulting in an exacerbated burn – may be an issue when citrus oils are applied topically. One must proceed with caution when applying essential oils using this method.

Inhalation Therapy

Commonly known as "aromatherapy," this essential oil application is effective for inner ailments, like sore throat or cold. In a steaming bowl of distilled, or sterilized water, add a few drops of essential oil and with a towel over your head, bend over the bowl and inhale. The towel captures the vapors making the technique even more effective. Essential oils can also be placed in a diffuser, or potpourri throughout a room, to produce somewhat diluted medicinal effects.

Ingestion

When using this method proceed with caution. Direct ingestion of essential oils must be monitored and applied in small doses that are diluted in a tablespoon or more of any carrier oil – olive oil, for example. If you are unsure of dosage amounts, then make a tea with the relevant herb instead. Although the effects of this diluted use may be weaker, this application is a better alternative than an overdose of essential oils.

What are the general benefits of using essential oils?

Replacement for Prescription Drugs

One practical benefit for using essential oils is their substitutive nature; they can replace Rx drugs, which is the ultimate reason to educate yourself on their administration and to begin stockpiling your essential oil supply. One of the potential threats of economic or social collapse, is the lack of resources, and primarily the inability to procure prescription drugs. As such, finding suitable alternatives should be a priority when prepping for the worst.

Their portability is also a major bonus when it comes to survival prepping. The fact that these ultra-concentrated oils take up little-to-no space makes toting them to your shelter all the easier should the need arise. Because essential oils are highly concentrated, the application used in most methods of administration requires only a drop or two of oil, which means a tiny bottle will be long-lasting.

Cheap, but Effective Alternative

Though money may be the last thing on your mind when it comes to prepping for a survival situation (money may even be obsolete in the event of social collapse), it is worth noting that the expense of essential oils pales in comparison to prescription drugs. In fact, whether or not you are forced to survive on essential oils due to a lack of prescription reserves, in some cases, you might consider substituting your prescriptions for these inexpensive alternatives regardless. Essential oils are a cost efficient, yet equally effective alternative to prescription medicine.

No Expiration Date

Another benefit of essential oils is that they do not expire, nor do they have "proper storage" requirements. A number of medicines and medicinal products must be replaced every couple years; this sets essential oils ahead of the pack when it comes to shelf life.

Versatility

Essential oils also offer great versatility. Apart from providing health benefits, essential oils can be repurposed for household and hygienic applications. For instance, if you are looking for something that might serve your dental hygiene needs in a time of crisis, thieves oil is your go-to essential oil. If you want to maintain your skin's health, frankincense and lavender will do the trick; the latter also serves as sunscreen, so you can prevent sun damage as well.

When it comes to the house or shelter you can use essential oils to deodorize, which will come in handy in a disaster scenario where things might start to smell due to lack of proper utilities and care. For example, after the 2011 tsunami and the subsequent nuclear reactor meltdown in Japan, a nurse named Risa Nakahira used essential oils to deodorize and sanitize putrid public bathrooms in overpopulated evacuation facilities. As relief workers searched for survivors, often wading through debris and decay, Nakahira also deodorized their boots and masks using essential oils. The possibilities of these natural oils are endless.

They are also versatile when it comes to the range of patients they are capable of supporting. The health of everyone from your great grandfather to your infant baby, can be fortified with the aid of essential oils in the appropriate dosage. They even come in handy when treating livestock or pets. From teething infants to dementia in the elderly, from teenagers with acne to dogs with urinary tract infections, essential oils can serve any patient with nearly any ailment.

Conclusion

Now that you know all about what lemon essential oil can do for you – where it originates, how it's extracted, its benefits and properties, and the different methods of administration – you can use it confidently to support the body's defenses against health issues and start to assemble a kit of essential oils for survival. Essential oils can be purchased online or at your local holistic treatment store. If you intend to stock up through online sources, you might try EverythingEssential.com or other like sites. We always recommend the brand guarantees high quality therapeutic grade oils that can be taken internally.

The various benefits of essential oils and their properties are countless. To build your own kit, first focus on acquiring the essential oils which may bear more relevance to your health issues or the potential health threats within your environment. In the event of a viral outbreak, for instance, lemon essential oil will be one of your more crucial oils – along with oregano, lemon, frankincense and cinnamon (eBooks also available for purchase) – due to their antiviral and immuno-supportive properties.

Used as a supplement or as your go-to for skin issues, viral infections or immune-boosting agents, the application of lemon essential oil in medicine has survived for centuries and will survive centuries more. When it comes down to it, you don't need to rely on pharmaceuticals; essential oils, herbs, and plenty of other natural ingredients can be used to help support the body's natural defenses against any number of health issues, whether ailment or injury.

Essential oils are essential to your survival in the case of viral outbreak, social collapse or natural disaster because, when the SHTF, your access to pharmaceuticals will likely either be limited or eliminated altogether. Alternatives to our modern-day standard will equate survival when no other option exists. And when it comes to a life-or-death situation, you can't let your health decline, no matter the state of the world.

DISCLAIMER AND/OR LEGAL NOTICES: Every effort has been made to accurately represent this book and it's potential. Results vary with every individual, and your results may or may not be different from those depicted. No promises, guarantees or warranties, whether stated or implied, have been made that you will produce any specific result from this book. Your efforts are individual and unique, and may vary from those shown. Your success depends on your efforts, background and motivation.

The material in this publication is provided for educational and informational purposes only and is not intended as medical advice. The information contained in this book should not be used to diagnose or treat any illness, metabolic disorder, disease or health problem. Always consult your physician or healthcare provider before beginning any nutrition or exercise program. Use of the programs, advice, and information contained in this book is at the sole choice and risk of the reader.